HOW TO HEAL PMS NATURALLY

How To Heal PMS

Naturally

JOHNSON WU

LOONS PRESS

How To Heal PMS Naturally

This publication is intended to provide educational information for the reader on the covered subjects. It is not intended to take the place of personalized medical counseling, diagnosis, and treatment from a trained healthcare professional.

ISBN 978-1-998455-83-6 (Paperback)
ISBN 978-1-998455-84-3 (eBook)

Printed and bound in USA
Published by Loons Press

Table Of Contents

Chapter 1

Understanding PMS

What is PMS?

PMS, or premenstrual syndrome, is a common condition that affects many people who menstruate. It refers to a combination of physical and emotional symptoms that occur in the days leading up to menstruation. These symptoms can vary widely from person to person and can range from mild to severe. While PMS is a normal part of the menstrual cycle for many individuals, it can be disruptive and uncomfortable for those who experience more severe symptoms.

The exact cause of PMS is not fully understood, but it is believed to be related to hormonal fluctuations that occur during the menstrual cycle. Changes in estrogen and progesterone levels can affect neurotransmitters in the brain, leading to mood swings, irritability, and other emotional symptoms. Additionally, changes in fluid retention and inflammation can cause physical symptoms such as bloating, breast tenderness, and fatigue.

It is important to note that PMS is not the same as PMDD, or premenstrual dysphoric disorder, which is a more severe form of PMS that can significantly impact a person's quality of life. While PMS symptoms are typically manageable with lifestyle changes and natural remedies, PMDD may require medical intervention and professional treatment.

Healing PMS holistically involves taking a comprehensive approach to managing symptoms and addressing the underlying causes of the condition. This may include making dietary changes, incorporating regular exercise, practicing stress-reducing techniques such as meditation or yoga, and using natural supplements to support hormone balance. By taking a holistic approach to healing PMS, individuals can better manage their symptoms and improve their overall well-being.

In conclusion, understanding what PMS is and how it affects the body is the first step in managing and healing the condition. By taking a holistic approach to addressing the physical and emotional symptoms of PMS, individuals can ind relief and improve their quality of life.

By incorporating natural remedies and lifestyle changes, those who experience PMS can empower themselves to take control of their health and well- being.

Common Symptoms of PMS

Many women experience premenstrual syndrome (PMS) symptoms at some point in their lives, with some experiencing more severe symptoms than others. Understanding the common symptoms of PMS can help you better manage and alleviate them. In this subchapter, we will discuss the most common symptoms of PMS and provide you with natural ways to heal and alleviate them holistically.

One of the most common symptoms of PMS is mood swings. Many women experience irritability, sadness, or anxiety in the days leading up to their period. These mood swings can be challenging to deal with but can be managed through various holistic approaches such as meditation, yoga, and deep breathing exercises. Additionally, making sure to get enough sleep, exercise regularly, and eat a healthy diet can also help stabilize your mood during this time.

Another common symptom of PMS is bloating and water retention. Many women experience a feeling of fullness or swelling in their abdomen, hands, and feet during this time.

To alleviate bloating naturally, try reducing your salt intake, drinking plenty of water, and eating foods that are high in potassium, such as bananas and leafy greens. Gentle exercises like walking or yoga can also help reduce bloating and water retention.

Fatigue and low energy levels are also common symptoms of PMS. Many women report feeling tired and lacking motivation in the days leading up to their period. To combat fatigue naturally, make sure to get enough rest, prioritize self-care activities, and eat a balanced diet rich in nutrients.

Regular exercise, such as brisk walking or gentle yoga, can also help boost your energy levels and improve your overall well-being during this time.

Cramps and abdominal pain are another common symptom of PMS that many women experience. These cramps can range from mild discomfort to severe pain and can be debilitating for some individuals. To alleviate cramps naturally, try using heat therapy, such as a heating pad or warm bath, to relax the muscles and reduce pain.

Gentle exercises like stretching or yoga poses can also help alleviate cramps and improve blood flow to the pelvic area, reducing discomfort.

In conclusion, understanding the common symptoms of PMS and how to heal them holistically can help you better manage your condition and improve your overall well-being. By incorporating natural remedies such as meditation, yoga, healthy eating, and self-care practices into your routine, you can alleviate PMS symptoms and feel more in control of your health and happiness.

Remember that every woman is different, and what works for one person may not work for another, so it's essential to experiment with different holistic approaches to ind what works best for you.

Causes of PMS

PMS, or premenstrual syndrome, is a common condition that affects many people who menstruate. While the exact cause of PMS is not fully understood, there are several factors that are believed to contribute to its development. One of the main causes of PMS is hormonal fluctuations.

During the menstrual cycle, levels of estrogen and progesterone rise and fall, which can lead to mood swings, irritability, and other symptoms commonly associated with PMS.

Another potential cause of PMS is imbalances in neurotransmitters, which are chemicals that help regulate mood and emotions. When these neurotransmitters are out of balance, it can lead to symptoms such as anxiety, depression, and irritability.

Additionally, some researchers believe that certain lifestyle factors, such as poor diet, lack of exercise, and high stress levels, can contribute to the development of PMS.

Diet can also play a significant role in the development of PMS. Consuming a diet high in processed foods, sugar, caffeine, and alcohol can exacerbate symptoms of PMS. These foods can lead to inflammation in the body, which can worsen symptoms such as bloating, cramps, and fatigue. On the other hand, a diet rich in fruits, vegetables, whole grains, and lean protein can help reduce inflammation and improve overall health, potentially alleviating symptoms of PMS.

In addition to hormonal fluctuations, neurotransmitter imbalances, and diet, other factors such as genetics and underlying health conditions can also contribute to the development of PMS. Some people may be more genetically predisposed to experiencing severe PMS symptoms, while others may have underlying health conditions such as thyroid disorders or polycystic ovary syndrome that can exacerbate symptoms.

It is important for individuals with PMS to work with a healthcare provider to address any underlying health conditions and develop a holistic treatment plan to manage symptoms.

In conclusion, PMS is a complex condition with multiple potential causes. By understanding the factors that contribute to the development of PMS, individuals can take steps to address these root causes and manage symptoms more effectively. Through lifestyle modifications, such as maintaining a healthy diet, exercising regularly, and managing stress, individuals can help alleviate symptoms of PMS and improve their overall quality of life.

Chapter 2

Holistic Approaches to Healing PMS

Diet and Nutrition

In this subchapter, we will explore the importance of diet and nutrition in managing and alleviating PMS symptoms. What we put into our bodies can have a significant impact on our overall health and well-being, including our hormonal balance. By making conscious choices about the foods we consume, we can support our bodies in achieving hormonal harmony and reducing the severity of PMS symptoms.

One of the key principles of a PMS-friendly diet is to focus on whole, nutrient-dense foods. This means choosing foods that are minimally processed and rich in vitamins, minerals, and antioxidants. By prioritizing fruits, vegetables, whole grains, lean proteins, and healthy fats, we can provide our bodies with the essential nutrients they need to function optimally and support hormonal balance.

It is also important to pay attention to the timing and frequency of meals. Eating regular, balanced meals throughout the day can help stabilize blood sugar levels and prevent energy crashes, mood swings, and cravings – all common symptoms of PMS. Aim to include a source of protein, healthy fats, and fiber in each meal to promote satiety and maintain steady energy levels.

In addition to choosing the right foods, it is important to be mindful of certain dietary triggers that may exacerbate PMS symptoms. For some individuals, consuming caffeine, alcohol, sugar, and processed foods can worsen symptoms such as bloating, irritability, and fatigue. Keeping a food diary can help you identify any potential triggers and make informed decisions about what to include or avoid in your diet.

Overall, taking a holistic approach to managing PMS through diet and nutrition can have a powerful impact on your overall well-being. By nourishing your body with nutrient-dense foods, balancing your meals, and being mindful of dietary triggers, you can support your hormonal balance and alleviate the symptoms of PMS naturally.

Remember that everyone is unique, so it may take some trial and error to ind the right approach for you. Consult with a healthcare provider or nutritionist for personalized guidance and support on your journey to healing PMS holistically.

Herbal Remedies

Herbal remedies have been used for centuries to alleviate the symptoms of PMS and provide relief to those who suffer from this condition. These natural remedies can be a safe and effective way to manage your symptoms without the need for harsh medications. In this subchapter, we will explore some of the most popular herbal remedies for PMS and how they can help you heal holistically.

One of the most well-known herbal remedies for PMS is chasteberry, also known as Vitex. This herb has been shown to help regulate hormone levels and reduce symptoms such as mood swings, bloating, and breast tenderness. By taking chasteberry regularly, you may experience a decrease in the severity of your PMS symptoms and an overall improvement in your well- being.

Another popular herbal remedy for PMS is evening primrose oil. This oil is rich in gamma- linolenic acid (GLA), which has anti-inflammatory properties that can help reduce cramping and breast pain associated with PMS. By incorporating evening primrose oil into your daily routine, you may ind relief from these uncomfortable symptoms and experience a greater sense of balance and calm during your menstrual cycle.

In addition to chasteberry and evening primrose oil, there are several other herbal remedies that can be beneficial for managing PMS symptoms. For example, dong quai is an herb that has been used in traditional Chinese medicine to help regulate menstrual cycles and alleviate symptoms of PMS. Similarly, black cohosh has been shown to reduce hot flashes, mood swings, and irritability in women experiencing PMS.

It is important to note that while herbal remedies can be effective for managing PMS symptoms, they may not work for everyone. It is always best to consult with a healthcare provider before starting any new herbal remedy to ensure it is safe and appropriate for your individual needs.

By incorporating herbal remedies into your holistic approach to healing PMS, you may ind relief from your symptoms and a greater sense of well-being during your menstrual cycle.

Stress Management Techniques

Stress management techniques are essential for individuals experiencing PMS symptoms. Stress can exacerbate hormonal imbalances and increase the severity of PMS symptoms. By incorporating stress management techniques into your daily routine, you can effectively alleviate some of the discomfort associated with PMS.

One effective stress management technique is deep breathing exercises. Deep breathing helps to calm the nervous system and reduce stress levels. Take a few moments each day to practice deep breathing by inhaling deeply through your nose, holding the breath for a few seconds, and then exhaling slowly through your mouth. This simple technique can help to reduce feelings of anxiety and tension.

Another helpful stress management technique is mindfulness meditation. Mindfulness meditation involves focusing on the present moment and accepting your thoughts and feelings without judgment.

By practicing mindfulness meditation regularly, you can cultivate a sense of calm and reduce stress levels. Consider setting aside a few minutes each day to practice mindfulness meditation and observe the positive impact it can have on your overall well-being.

Physical activity is also an important stress management technique for individuals experiencing PMS symptoms. Exercise releases endorphins, which are natural mood boosters that can help to alleviate stress and improve your overall mood. Engaging in regular physical activity, such as walking, yoga, or swimming, can help to reduce stress levels and improve your overall well-being.

Incorporating stress management techniques into your daily routine can help you effectively manage the symptoms of PMS and improve your overall quality of life. By practicing deep breathing exercises, mindfulness meditation, and engaging in regular physical activity, you can reduce stress levels, alleviate PMS symptoms, and promote a sense of well-being. Take the time to prioritize your mental and emotional health by incorporating these stress management techniques into your daily routine.

Chapter 3

Creating a Holistic Healing Plan

Identifying Triggers

Identifying triggers is a crucial step in effectively managing PMS symptoms. By recognizing what factors contribute to your discomfort, you can take proactive steps to address them and minimize their impact on your well-being. Triggers can vary from person to person, so it's important to pay attention to your own body and emotions to pinpoint what may be exacerbating your symptoms.

One common trigger for PMS is stress. When we experience high levels of stress, our bodies release cortisol, a hormone that can disrupt the delicate balance of other hormones involved in the menstrual cycle. To combat this, it's important to ind healthy ways to manage stress, such as practicing relaxation techniques like deep breathing, meditation, or yoga. Additionally, getting regular exercise and prioritizing self-care can help reduce stress levels and improve overall well-being.

Another trigger for PMS is diet. Certain foods, such as those high in sugar, caffeine, or processed ingredients, can worsen symptoms like bloating, mood swings, and fatigue. Keeping a food diary can help you identify which foods may be triggering your symptoms so you can make informed choices about what to eat. Incorporating more whole, nutrient-rich foods like fruits, vegetables, whole grains, and lean proteins can help support hormone balance and alleviate PMS symptoms.

Hormonal fluctuations are also a common trigger for PMS. Changes in estrogen and progesterone levels throughout the menstrual cycle can impact mood, energy levels, and physical symptoms.

Tracking your menstrual cycle can help you identify when these hormonal shifts occur and when you may be more susceptible to experiencing PMS symptoms. This can empower you to anticipate and prepare for potential triggers, such as by adjusting your schedule or prioritizing self-care during vulnerable times.

Environmental factors, such as exposure to toxins or allergens, can also play a role in triggering PMS symptoms. Pay attention to your surroundings and any changes that may coincide with the onset of your symptoms. Making simple adjustments, such as using natural cleaning products, avoiding known allergens, or spending more time outdoors in fresh air, can help reduce your overall toxic load and minimize potential triggers for PMS.

By identifying and addressing triggers, you can take a proactive approach to managing your PMS symptoms holistically and improving your overall quality of life.

Developing a Self-Care Routine

Developing a self-care routine is crucial for managing PMS symptoms and promoting overall well- being. By incorporating self-care practices into your daily routine, you can help alleviate the physical and emotional discomfort that often accompanies PMS. In this subchapter, we will explore various self-care strategies that can help you heal PMS holistically and improve your quality of life.

One important aspect of developing a self-care routine for PMS is paying attention to your body's needs. This includes getting enough rest, eating a balanced diet, and engaging in regular physical activity. Adequate sleep is essential for hormone regulation and mood stability, so be sure to prioritize restful sleep by establishing a consistent bedtime routine and creating a peaceful sleep environment. Additionally, consuming nutrient-rich foods and staying hydrated can help support your body's natural hormone balance and reduce PMS symptoms.

Incorporating stress-reducing activities into your daily routine can also be beneficial for managing PMS symptoms. Chronic stress can exacerbate hormonal imbalances and increase the severity of PMS symptoms, so it's important to ind healthy ways to cope with stress.

Meditation, deep breathing exercises, yoga, and journaling are all effective techniques for relieving stress and promoting relaxation. By incorporating these practices into your daily routine, you can help reduce the impact of stress on your physical and emotional well-being.

Another key component of a self-care routine for PMS is prioritizing self-care activities that bring you joy and relaxation. Engaging in activities that you enjoy, whether it's reading a book, taking a bath, or spending time in nature, can help boost your mood and reduce PMS symptoms.

Making time for self-care activities is essential for maintaining a positive mindset and promoting emotional well-being during the challenging time of the month.

In conclusion, developing a self-care routine is an essential aspect of healing PMS holistically and improving your overall quality of life. By paying attention to your body's needs, incorporating stress- reducing activities, and prioritizing self-care activities that bring you joy and relaxation, you can effectively manage PMS symptoms and promote emotional well- being.

Remember that self-care is not selfish – it is a necessary part of maintaining your health and well- being, especially during times of hormonal imbalance like PMS.

Seeking Professional Help

If you have been struggling with the symptoms of PMS and have not found relief through natural remedies and lifestyle changes, it may be time to seek professional help. A healthcare provider, such as a gynecologist can help you navigate your symptoms and provide personalized treatment options to help you manage your PMS more effectively.

When seeking professional help for PMS, it is important to be prepared for your appointment. Keep a detailed record of your symptoms, including when they occur and how they impact your daily life. This information can help your healthcare provider better understand your condition and tailor a treatment plan to address your specific needs.

During your appointment, be open and honest about your symptoms and how they are affecting you. Your healthcare provider may recommend further testing to rule out any underlying medical conditions that could be contributing to your PMS symptoms. They may also suggest lifestyle changes, dietary modifications, or natural supplements to help alleviate your symptoms.

In some cases, your healthcare provider may recommend medications to help manage your PMS symptoms. These may include nonsteroidal anti- inflammatory drugs (NSAIDs) for pain relief, hormonal contraceptives to regulate your menstrual cycle, or antidepressants to help with mood swings and anxiety. Your healthcare provider will work with you to ind the best treatment plan for your individual needs.

Remember, seeking professional help for your PMS does not mean that you have failed in your efforts to heal holistically. It simply means that you are taking proactive steps to address your symptoms and improve your quality of life. By working with a healthcare provider, you can gain valuable insights and support to help you manage your PMS more effectively and ind relief from your symptoms.

Chapter 4

Implementing Lifestyle Changes

Exercise and Physical Activity

Exercise and physical activity play a crucial role in managing and alleviating the symptoms of premenstrual syndrome (PMS). Regular exercise has been shown to improve mood, reduce stress, and increase energy levels, all of which are important factors in combating the physical and emotional symptoms of PMS.

By incorporating exercise into your daily routine, you can help regulate your hormone levels, improve circulation, and boost your overall well-being.

When it comes to choosing the right type of exercise for managing PMS, it's important to ind activities that you enjoy and that it your individual needs and preferences.

Whether it's yoga, walking, swimming, or strength training, the key is to ind something that you can stick to and that helps you feel good both mentally and physically. Aim for at least 30 minutes of moderate exercise most days of the week to experience the full benefits of physical activity on your PMS symptoms.

In addition to helping with mood regulation and stress reduction, exercise can also help alleviate physical symptoms associated with PMS, such as bloating, cramps, and breast tenderness. By engaging in regular physical activity, you can improve your muscle tone, flexibility, and overall strength, which can help reduce the severity of these physical symptoms. Furthermore, exercise has been shown to release endorphins, the body's natural feel-good chemicals, which can help reduce pain and discomfort during your menstrual cycle.

It's important to listen to your body and adjust your exercise routine accordingly during different phases of your menstrual cycle. While some women may ind that high-intensity workouts are beneficial during certain times of the month, others may prefer more gentle forms of exercise, such as restorative yoga or walking, during their period.

By tuning into your body's signals and adjusting your exercise routine accordingly, you can maximize the benefits of physical activity on your PMS symptoms.

In conclusion, incorporating regular exercise and physical activity into your routine can have a significant impact on managing and alleviating the symptoms of PMS. By finding activities that you enjoy and that it your individual needs, you can improve your mood, reduce stress, alleviate physical symptoms, and boost your overall well-being. Remember to listen to your body and adjust your exercise routine as needed throughout your menstrual cycle to optimize the benefits of physical activity on your PMS symptoms.

Sleep Hygiene

Sleep hygiene is an essential aspect of managing PMS symptoms naturally. Quality sleep is crucial for hormone regulation, mood stability, and overall well- being. Establishing good sleep hygiene practices can help alleviate PMS symptoms and improve your quality of life. In this subchapter, we will explore the importance of sleep hygiene and provide practical tips to help you get a restful night's sleep.

First and foremost, it is important to maintain a consistent sleep schedule. Going to bed and waking up at the same time every day helps regulate your body's internal clock and promote better sleep. Avoiding caffeine, alcohol, and heavy meals close to bedtime can also improve your sleep quality. These substances can disrupt your sleep patterns and make it harder to fall asleep or stay asleep throughout the night.

Creating a relaxing bedtime routine can signal to your body that it is time to wind down and prepare for sleep. Engaging in calming activities such as reading, meditating, or taking a warm bath can help reduce stress and promote relaxation. It is also important to create a comfortable sleep environment by keeping your bedroom dark, quiet, and cool. Investing in a supportive mattress and pillows can also improve your sleep quality.

Limiting screen time before bed is another important aspect of sleep hygiene. The blue light emitted by electronic devices can disrupt your body's production of melatonin, a hormone that regulates sleep-wake cycles.

Try to avoid using screens at least an hour before bedtime and consider using blue light blocking glasses or apps to reduce your exposure to blue light. Instead, opt for activities that promote relaxation and prepare your body for sleep.

In conclusion, prioritizing sleep hygiene is crucial for managing PMS symptoms naturally. By establishing a consistent sleep schedule, creating a relaxing bedtime routine, and limiting screen time before bed, you can improve your sleep quality and alleviate PMS symptoms. Remember that good sleep is essential for hormone regulation, mood stability, and overall well-being. By implementing these tips into your daily routine, you can support your body's natural healing process and improve your quality of life.

Mind-Body Practices

Mind-body practices are an essential component in healing PMS naturally. These practices involve connecting the mind and body to promote overall well- being and balance. By incorporating techniques such as meditation, yoga, and deep breathing exercises into your daily routine, you can help alleviate the symptoms of PMS and improve your overall quality of life.

Meditation is a powerful tool for calming the mind and reducing stress, which can exacerbate PMS symptoms. By taking a few minutes each day to sit quietly and focus on your breath, you can cultivate a sense of inner peace and relaxation. This can help to reduce anxiety, mood swings, and irritability that often accompany PMS.

Additionally, meditation can help improve sleep quality, which is essential for managing PMS symptoms.

Yoga is another effective mind-body practice for healing PMS holistically. The gentle stretching and strengthening exercises in yoga can help improve circulation, reduce muscle tension, and promote relaxation.

Certain yoga poses, such as child's pose and cat- cow pose, can specifically target the areas of the body that are most affected by PMS, such as the lower back and abdomen. Regular yoga practice can also help regulate hormonal imbalances and improve overall hormonal health.

Deep breathing exercises are another valuable tool for relieving PMS symptoms. By focusing on slow, deep breaths, you can activate the body's relaxation response and reduce symptoms such as bloating, headaches, and fatigue. Deep breathing can also help calm the nervous system and improve mood, making it a valuable practice for managing the emotional ups and downs of PMS. Incorporating deep breathing exercises into your daily routine can help you feel more grounded and centered during the challenging days of your menstrual cycle.

Overall, mind-body practices are a powerful and natural way to heal PMS holistically. By incorporating practices such as meditation, yoga, and deep breathing exercises into your daily routine, you can help alleviate the physical and emotional symptoms of PMS and improve your overall well-being. These practices can help you feel more in tune with your body and mind, leading to a greater sense of balance and harmony during your menstrual cycle.

Chapter 5

Tracking Progress and Adjusting Your Plan

Keeping a Symptom Journal

Keeping a symptom journal is a crucial tool for anyone looking to heal PMS naturally. By recording your symptoms on a daily basis, you can gain valuable insights into your body's patterns and triggers. This information can help you identify specific changes you can make to improve your symptoms and overall well- being.

Start by creating a simple chart or diary where you can track your PMS symptoms each day. Include details such as the date, time, severity, duration, and any potential triggers or factors that may have contributed to your symptoms. This will help you see patterns over time and make connections between your symptoms and your lifestyle choices.

When keeping a symptom journal, it's important to be as detailed and honest as possible. Don't be afraid to write down even the smallest changes or symptoms you experience. This information can be invaluable in helping you and your healthcare provider understand your unique PMS experience and tailor a treatment plan that works best for you.

Reviewing your symptom journal regularly can also help you identify any progress or setbacks in your healing journey. By tracking your symptoms over time, you can see if certain lifestyle changes or treatments are helping to alleviate your PMS symptoms. This information can empower you to make informed decisions about your health and make adjustments as needed.

Overall, keeping a symptom journal is a proactive way to take control of your PMS symptoms and work towards healing holistically. By documenting your experiences and patterns, you can better understand your body's needs and make positive changes that support your overall well-being. So grab a notebook and start recording your symptoms today – your body will thank you for it!

Evaluating Your Healing Plan

Once you have developed a holistic healing plan for your PMS symptoms, it is important to regularly evaluate its effectiveness. By assessing how well your plan is working, you can make necessary adjustments to ensure you are on the right track towards healing PMS naturally.

One way to evaluate your healing plan is to keep a detailed journal of your symptoms and any changes you have made to your lifestyle or diet. By tracking your symptoms over time, you can identify patterns and determine what is working well and what may need to be adjusted. This can help you pinpoint triggers for your PMS and make informed decisions about how to best manage your symptoms.

It is also important to regularly check in with your healthcare provider or holistic practitioner to discuss your progress and any changes you have noticed. They can provide valuable insight and guidance on how to further optimize your healing plan. Additionally, they may recommend additional therapies or treatments that can support your holistic approach to healing PMS.

In evaluating your healing plan, it is essential to be patient and persistent. Healing PMS naturally is a journey that takes time and dedication. By staying committed to your plan and being open to making changes as needed, you can achieve long-lasting relief from your symptoms and improve overall well-being.

Remember, healing PMS holistically is a personalized process that requires self-awareness and a willingness to experiment with different approaches. By regularly evaluating your healing plan and making adjustments as needed, you can empower yourself to take control of your health and live a life free from the burden of PMS.

Making Necessary Adjustments

Making necessary adjustments is a crucial step in healing PMS naturally. By identifying the root causes of your symptoms and making lifestyle changes, you can effectively manage and reduce the severity of your PMS. It is important to remember that everyone's body is different, so what works for one person may not work for another. It may take some trial and error to ind the right combination of adjustments that work best for you.

One key adjustment to make is to focus on your diet. Certain foods can exacerbate PMS symptoms, such as processed foods, caffeine, alcohol, and sugary treats. By incorporating more whole foods, such as fruits, vegetables, whole grains, and lean proteins, you can help balance your hormones and reduce inflammation in the body.

Additionally, staying hydrated and avoiding excess salt can help alleviate bloating and water retention commonly associated with PMS.

Another important adjustment to consider is managing stress. Chronic stress can worsen PMS symptoms by increasing cortisol levels and disrupting hormone balance. Incorporating stress-reducing activities into your daily routine, such as yoga, meditation, deep breathing exercises, or spending time in nature, can help calm your nervous system and improve your overall well-being. Prioritizing self-care and setting boundaries with work and relationships can also help reduce stress levels.

Regular exercise is another vital adjustment to make when healing PMS naturally. Physical activity can help reduce PMS symptoms by releasing endorphins, improving circulation, and balancing hormones. Aim for at least 30 minutes of moderate exercise most days of the week, such as walking, biking, swimming, or yoga. Find activities that you enjoy and make them a regular part of your routine to help manage your PMS symptoms effectively.

In addition to these lifestyle adjustments, it may be beneficial to explore natural supplements and herbs that can support hormone balance and reduce PMS symptoms. Vitex, magnesium, evening primrose oil, and omega-3 fatty acids are commonly used to alleviate PMS symptoms. However, it is important to consult with a healthcare provider before starting any new supplements to ensure they are safe and appropriate for your individual needs.

By making these necessary adjustments and taking a holistic approach to healing PMS, you can empower yourself to manage your symptoms and improve your quality of life.

Chapter 6

Resources for Continued Support

Online Communities and Support Groups

Online communities and support groups can be invaluable resources for individuals dealing with PMS. These platforms provide a safe space for people to share their experiences, offer advice, and seek support from others who understand what they are going through. Connecting with like-minded individuals can help alleviate feelings of isolation and provide a sense of belonging.

One of the key benefits of online communities and support groups is the wealth of information available at your fingertips. From natural remedies to holistic approaches to managing PMS symptoms, you can ind a wide range of resources to help you navigate your journey towards healing. By tapping into the collective wisdom of the community, you can discover new strategies and techniques that may work for you.

In addition to practical advice, online communities and support groups offer emotional support and encouragement. Dealing with PMS can be emotionally taxing, and having a group of people who understand and empathize with your struggles can make a world of difference. Whether you need a listening ear, a virtual hug, or words of encouragement, these communities can provide the emotional support you need to stay strong and resilient.

Furthermore, online communities and support groups can help you stay motivated and accountable on your healing journey. By setting goals, sharing your progress, and celebrating your successes with others, you can stay on track and continue moving forward towards optimal health. The sense of camaraderie and shared purpose within these groups can be incredibly empowering and motivating.

In conclusion, online communities and support groups can be powerful tools for individuals seeking to heal PMS holistically. By connecting with others who share similar experiences and goals, you can access a wealth of information, emotional support, and motivation to help you on your journey towards healing.

Whether you are looking for practical advice, emotional support, or accountability, these communities can provide the resources you need to thrive.

Recommended Books and Websites

In the journey to healing PMS naturally, it is essential to equip yourself with resources that will empower and guide you towards holistic well-being. This subchapter, "Recommended Books and Websites," aims to provide valuable information for individuals experiencing PMS. By delving into the wealth of knowledge available in these recommended books and websites, you can gain insights, strategies, and tools to effectively manage and alleviate your PMS symptoms.

One highly recommended book for individuals dealing with PMS is "The Period Repair Manual" by Dr. Lara Briden. This comprehensive guide offers practical advice on understanding your menstrual cycle, identifying hormonal imbalances, and implementing natural remedies to address PMS symptoms.

Dr. Briden's evidence-based approach and wealth of experience make this book a valuable resource for anyone seeking to heal PMS holistically.

Another valuable resource for individuals navigating PMS is the website HormonesBalance.com. Founded by holistic nutritionist Magdalena Wszelaki, this website provides a wealth of information on how to balance hormones naturally, including specific strategies for managing PMS symptoms. From dietary recommendations to lifestyle tips, HormonesBalance.com offers practical tools and resources to support your journey towards hormonal health and well-being.

For individuals seeking a deeper understanding of the mind-body connection in relation to PMS, the book "Women's Bodies, Women's Wisdom" by Dr. Christiane Northrup is an invaluable resource. Dr. Northrup explores the intricate relationship between emotions, stress, and hormonal health, offering insights into how our thoughts and feelings impact our physical well- being. By incorporating the wisdom shared in this book, individuals can gain a holistic perspective on healing PMS from a mind-body-spirit approach.

In addition to these recommended resources, it is important to explore and discover other books and websites that resonate with your unique journey towards healing PMS holistically. By immersing yourself in knowledge, insights, and practical strategies from trusted sources, you can empower yourself to take charge of your hormonal health and well-being. Remember, knowledge is power, and by arming yourself with valuable resources, you can embark on a transformative journey towards healing PMS naturally and holistically.

Finding a Holistic Healthcare Provider

When seeking to heal PMS holistically, finding a healthcare provider who aligns with your values and beliefs is essential. A holistic healthcare provider takes into account the whole person - mind, body, and spirit - when creating a treatment plan. This approach can be highly beneficial for those with PMS, as it addresses the root causes of symptoms rather than just treating them superficially. Here are some tips for finding a holistic healthcare provider who can help you on your journey to healing PMS naturally.

First and foremost, it is important to do your research when looking for a holistic healthcare provider. Look for practitioners who specialize in women's health and have experience treating PMS specifically. You may want to consider seeking out a naturopathic doctor, functional medicine practitioner, or holistic nutritionist who can offer a comprehensive approach to treating your symptoms.

When meeting with a potential healthcare provider, be sure to ask about their approach to treating PMS. A good holistic practitioner will take the time to listen to your concerns, ask detailed questions about your symptoms and health history, and work with you to create a personalized treatment plan. They may recommend dietary changes, supplements, herbal remedies, stress-reducing techniques, and other natural therapies to help alleviate your PMS symptoms.

It is also important to consider the location and accessibility of the healthcare provider. Choose someone who is conveniently located and easy to reach, as you may need to visit them regularly for follow-up appointments or treatment sessions.

Additionally, consider whether the provider accepts your insurance or offers payment plans to make treatment more affordable.

Another important factor to consider when choosing a holistic healthcare provider is their credentials and experience. Look for practitioners who are licensed and have advanced training in their field. You may also want to ask for references or read reviews from other patients to ensure that the provider has a good reputation and track record of success in treating PMS naturally.

Overall, finding a holistic healthcare provider who can help you heal PMS naturally is an important step in your journey to better health. By taking the time to research, ask questions, and choose a provider who aligns with your values and beliefs, you can set yourself up for success in managing your PMS symptoms and improving your overall well-being.

Chapter 7

Conclusion

Reflecting on Your Healing Journey

As you continue on your journey to healing PMS holistically, it is important to take time to reflect on how far you have come. Acknowledge the progress you have made, no matter how small it may seem. Reflecting on your healing journey can help you stay motivated and focused on your goals. It can also help you identify any areas where you may need to make adjustments or seek additional support.

Take some time to journal about your experiences with PMS and the changes you have implemented in your life to address it. Reflect on how these changes have impacted your symptoms and overall well-being. Consider keeping a symptom diary to track your progress and identify any patterns that may be helpful in managing your symptoms.

Reflecting on your healing journey can also help you celebrate your successes. Take note of any improvements in your symptoms, mood, energy levels, or quality of life. Celebrate these victories, no matter how small they may seem. Recognizing and celebrating your progress can boost your confidence and motivation to continue on your path to healing.

In addition to celebrating your successes, it is also important to acknowledge any setbacks or challenges you may have faced along the way. Reflect on what may have triggered these setbacks and consider what you can do differently in the future to prevent them from occurring again. Remember that setbacks are a natural part of the healing process and can provide valuable insights for growth and learning.

Overall, reflecting on your healing journey is an important part of the healing process. It can help you stay motivated, celebrate your successes, and learn from any setbacks you may encounter. By taking the time to reflect on your experiences, you can continue to make progress towards healing PMS holistically and achieving a greater sense of well-being.

Celebrating Your Progress

Congratulations! You have taken the first step towards healing your PMS naturally. It is important to celebrate your progress along this journey as you work towards finding relief from your symptoms. Each milestone, no matter how small, is a step in the right direction towards achieving optimal health and well- being. By acknowledging and celebrating your progress, you are reinforcing positive behaviors and empowering yourself to continue on this path towards healing.

One way to celebrate your progress is by keeping a journal to track your symptoms and the changes you have made in your lifestyle. Take note of any improvements you have noticed, whether it be a reduction in pain, increased energy levels, or improved mood.

Reflecting on these positive changes can help you stay motivated and committed to your holistic healing journey. It is also a great way to see how far you have come and remind yourself of the progress you have made.

Another way to celebrate your progress is by treating yourself to something special when you reach a specific goal. This could be a relaxing spa day, a new book, or a healthy meal at your favorite restaurant. Rewarding yourself for your hard work and dedication can help boost your morale and keep you motivated to continue making positive changes in your life.

Remember, self-care is an essential part of healing PMS holistically, so treat yourself with kindness and compassion.

Celebrate your progress by sharing your journey with others who may be experiencing similar challenges. Joining a support group or online community of people who have PMS can provide you with a sense of belonging and camaraderie.

Sharing your successes and challenges with others can help you feel less alone and more supported on your healing journey. It can also inspire and motivate others to take control of their health and well- being.

In conclusion, celebrating your progress is an important part of healing PMS holistically. By acknowledging your achievements, rewarding yourself for your hard work, and sharing your journey with others, you can stay motivated and inspired to continue making positive changes in your life.

Remember, healing is a journey, not a destination, so be kind to yourself and celebrate each step you take towards achieving optimal health and well-being.

Moving Forward with Confidence

Moving forward with confidence is an essential step in the journey to healing PMS naturally. It is important to understand that managing PMS holistically is a process that requires dedication and commitment.

By taking control of your health and well-being, you can empower yourself to make positive changes that will have a lasting impact on your symptoms.

One of the first steps in moving forward with confidence is to educate yourself about PMS and the various holistic approaches to treatment. By arming yourself with knowledge, you can make informed decisions about your health and well-being. Understanding the root causes of PMS and how they can be addressed through natural remedies and lifestyle changes is crucial to finding long-term relief.

In addition to educating yourself, it is important to develop a personalized plan for managing your PMS symptoms. This plan should include a combination of dietary changes, herbal supplements, stress management techniques, and regular exercise. By taking a holistic approach to treatment, you can address the underlying imbalances in your body that are contributing to your symptoms.

As you begin to implement your personalized plan for managing PMS, it is important to be patient and consistent. Healing holistically takes time, and it is important to give your body the opportunity to respond to the changes you are making. By staying committed to your plan and making adjustments as needed, you can make steady progress towards healing PMS naturally.

Moving forward with confidence means believing in your ability to overcome PMS and reclaim your health and well-being. By taking a proactive approach to managing your symptoms and staying focused on your goals, you can achieve lasting relief from PMS and enjoy a greater sense of vitality and well-being. Remember, you have the power to heal yourself holistically – trust in your body's ability to heal and embrace the journey ahead with confidence.

Author Notes & Acknowledgments

First and foremost, I would like to express my deepest gratitude to the people who inspired and supported me throughout the journey of writing this book. This project would not have been possible without their unwavering belief in me and their invaluable contributions.

To my wife, thank you for your constant encouragement and understanding. Your love and support have been my anchor during the challenging times of researching and writing this book. Your belief in my ability to make a difference in people's lives has been my driving force.

I would also like to disclose that this book contains some renewed artificial intelligence- generated content. I really appreciate very recent technological innovation by outstanding scientists and of course our reader's understanding.

Lastly, I want to express my deepest gratitude to the readers of this book. I sincerely hope the strategies and methods outlined within these pages will provide you with the knowledge and tools needed to truly make your life much better. Your commitment to seeking any good solutions and willingness to explore multiple methods is commendable.

Author Bio

Johnson Wu earned his MD in 1982. With over 40 years of clinical experience, he has worked in hospitals in Zhejiang and Shanghai, China, as well as the Royal Marsden Hospital (part of Imperial College) in London, UK.

Upon the recommendation of Sir Aaron Klug, the president of The Royal Society and a Nobel Prize winner in Chemistry, Dr. Wu was honorably awarded a British Royal Society Fellowship. He has published medical books and articles in seven countries and currently practices medicine in Canada.

www.ingramcontent.com/pod-product-compliance
Lightning Source LLC
Chambersburg PA
CBHW071036050426
42335CB00050B/1796